Practice SBA
Primary FRCA

Simon A. May

CONTENTS

INTRODUCTION

At the time of writing, the MCQ component of the Primary FRCA examination comprises 90 multiple choice questions, to be completed within 3 hours. 30 of these questions are single best answer (SBA) questions and the remaining 60 questions are multiple true/false (MTF) questions. The MTF questions are designed to test theoretical knowledge, whereas the SBA questions will require you to apply this knowledge.

Due to the weight of marks that the SBA questions carry (4 marks for each correct answer), the SBA section of the exam often proves to be a stumbling block to successful progression. This book contains 90 SBA questions, arranged into 3 practice papers. The MTF components of the Primary FRCA MCQ exam are covered in separate books in the *Revise Anaesthesia* series.

In contrast to MTF questions, a well written SBA question should contain more than one plausible answer. However, it is unlikely that all answers will be equally plausible, so it should be possible to narrow down the correct answer to a couple of possibilities. All of the questions have been written in a style that is similar to the questions you will face in the FRCA examinations and for each question, there is a concise explanation.

MCQ books are an essential aid to FRCA exam revision. They quickly identify gaps in knowledge and therefore help focus future revision. The *Revise Anaesthesia* series differs from other MCQ books, as you are able to purchase questions separately for each component of the exam. This allows the books to be used as part of topic-specific revision and provides an alternative to expensive subscription-based question banks.

Available in paperback and e-book format, the questions are yours to keep and access anywhere.

Best of luck in the examinations.

Paper 1

Q1:

A new anaesthetic agent has a boiling point of 56.5°C, a saturated vapour pressure of 175kPa at 20°C, a molecular weight of 184, a blood:gas coefficient of 1.91 and an oil:gas coefficient of 98.5. Which one of the following statements is true?

    A. It will require an injection vaporiser for safe use
    B. It is less potent than sevoflurane
    C. It has a slower onset than halothane
    D. It has the same molecular weight as isoflurane
    E. The minimum alveolar concentration (MAC) value will be less than isoflurane

Q2:

You are investigating the electrical potential across a squid axon and have decided to take into account all the ions that are present in the intra and extracellular space. Which equation should be utilised to derive the correct value?

    A. Application of Goldman equation
    B. Application of Nernst equation
    C. Application of van't Hoff equation
    D. Application of Gibbs-Donnan effect
    E. Application of Stewart's strong ion theorem

Q3:

A farmer presents to the accident and emergency department with hyper salivation, lacrimation and diarrhoea. He then progresses to muscle weakness with fasciculation and seizures which require intubation. Which of the following medications should be administered?

    A. Ecothiopate
    B. Pyridostigmine
    C. Pralidoxime
    D. Intralipid
    E. Neostigmine

Q4:

You are commencing a variable rate insulin infusion (VRII) on a type II diabetic patient due to undergo major abdominal surgery. Which fluid should be prescribed to run alongside the VRII?

    A. 5% glucose
    B. 5% glucose in 0.45% saline with 0.15% potassium
    C. 4% glucose in 0.18% saline with 0.15% potassium
    D. Alternate 5% glucose with 0.9% saline
    E. No intravenous fluid is required with VRII

Q5:

A patient is suffering from orthostatic hypotension and is prescribed a medication to act as a vasopressive agent. It is a racemix solution that is a prodrug with the active metabolite binding to the alpha-1 adrenergic receptor. It has no beta adrenergic activity and does not cross the blood-brain barrier. It has a bioavailability of 93% and is a colourless and odourless chemical. Which agent is being prescribed?

A. Noradrenaline
B. Methyl-dopa
C. Midodrine
D. Reserpine
E. Vasopressin

Q6:

A patient has been receiving heparin for an ischaemic limb caused by peripheral vascular disease. He has had repeated boluses of intravenous unfractionated heparin and a heparin infusion, but his APTT ratio remains sub-therapeutic. In the recent past he has had a prolonged course of intravenous unfractionated heparin. What is the likely cause for the sub-therapeutic APTT ratio?

A) Heparin induced thrombocytopaenia
B) Protein C deficiency
C) Protein S deficiency
D) Anti thrombin III deficiency
E) Hypercalcaemic state

Q7:

A patient is intubated and ventilated on intensive care after being admitted with shortness of breath. He has a blood pressure of 70/40mmHg, heart rate 120bpm, central venous pressure 20mmHg and a pulmonary capillary wedge pressure of 25mmHg. He has a PaO_2 of 8kPa on an FiO_2 of 1.0. What is the likely diagnosis?

    A. Pulmonary oedema
    B. Acute Respiratory Distress Syndrome (ARDS)
    C. Cardiac tamponade
    D. Pneumonia
    E. Anaphylaxis

Q8:

An 85 year old gentleman undergoes uneventful intramedullary nailing of a femoral shaft fracture with bone cement under spinal anaesthetic. In recovery he is hypotensive, tachycardic, pale and tachypnoeic despite saturating 100% on the pulse oximeter. What is the likely aetiology?

    A. Hypovolaemia due to blood loss
    B. Bone cement implantation syndrome
    C. Fat embolism
    D. Anaphylaxis
    E. Pulmonary embolism

Q9:

A 25 year old adult presents to hospital after sustaining chemical burn injuries after being sprayed by an unknown substance. He has bilateral circumferential leg burns and his groin, anterior abdomen and anterior chest show the stigmata of burn injury. Approximately how much of his body surface is burnt?

    A. 28%
    B. 37%
    C. 46%
    D. 55%
    E. 82%

Q10:

An epidural for caesarean section is "topped up" with 20mls of 2% lignocaine and 100mcg of fentanyl. Shortly afterwards the woman becomes agitated and then looses consciousness. She then develops a bradycardia and suffers a tonic-clonic seizure. She has a past history of epilepsy and her pregnancy was complicated by pregnancy-induced hypertension. She is 60Kg and has a height of 1.5m. What is the most likely diagnosis?

    A. Eclamptic seizure
    B. Local anaesthetic toxicity
    C. Total spinal
    D. Subdural catheter placement
    E. Anaphylaxis

Q11:

A 25 year old male has been involved in a road traffic accident as a pedestrian. He is brought to accident and emergency and is found to have a heart rate of 45bpm, blood pressure of 75/30mmHg, flaccid lower limb weakness, no anal tone, warm lower limbs, and absent reflexes of the lower limbs. What is the likely diagnosis?

A. Transection of the spinal cord at T6
B. Transection of the spinal cord at T1
C. Transection of the spinal cord at C2
D. Brown-Sequard syndrome
E. Anterior spinal artery syndrome

Q12:

Non-parametric data has been obtained from a study and demonstrates a positive kurtosis. Which statement is correct?

A. The value of the mode is higher than the median which is higher than the mean
B. The value of the mean is higher than the median which is higher than the mode
C. The value of the median is higher than the mode which is higher than the mean
D. The value of the mean is higher than the mode which is higher than the median
E. The mean, median and mode are the same

Q13:

A patient with myasthenia gravis undergoes laparotomy for a perforated sigmoid colon. At the end of the procedure she has no twitches on train-of-four monitoring. She was given thiopentone 400mg and suxamethonium 200mg at induction. She was given a single dose of actracurium 20mg, 200mcg fentanyl and morphine 10mg. 320mg gentamicin and co-amoxiclav 1.2g were also given. She was slightly hyperkalaemic and hypercalcaemic at induction of anaesthesia. Which of the following is likely to have delayed her recovery from neuromuscular blockade?

A. 200mg suxamethonium
B. 200mcg fentanyl
C. 320mg gentamicin
D. Hyperkalaemia
E. Hypercalcaemia

Q14:

A patient with malignant hypertension is admitted to intensive care and commenced on a sodium nitroprusside infusion. He has left ventricular enlargement, renal impairment with an eGFR $10\text{mlmin}^{-1}1.73\text{m}^{-2}$, visual changes and headache. Over the course of the night he develops a pH of 7.1 and base excess of -15mEql^{-1} from previously normal results. What is the likely aetiology?

A. Progression of renal dysfunction
B. Infarction of the pituitary gland
C. Aortic dissection
D. Myocardial infarction
E. Cyanide toxicity

Q15:

A 69 year old gentleman presents with acute onset of shortness of breath and chest pain. He is noted to have cannon A waves on his central venous waveform and a central venous pressure of 15mmHg. He has a heart rate of 150bpm measured at the radial artery and his blood pressure is 70/40mmHg. What is the likely aetiology:

A. Cardiac tamponade
B. Aortic dissection
C. Pulmonary embolism
D. Complete heart block
E. Atrio-ventricular nodal re-entrant tachycardia

Q16:

You are investigating the total body water of a student volunteer. Which is the appropriate biomarker for the experiment?

A. Antipyrine
B. Radioisotope of sodium
C. Radioisotope of albumin
D. Radioisotope of mannitol
E. radioisotope of chloride

Q17:

A patient presents to accident and emergency with a head injury. His eyes open to pain, he is making incomprehensible sounds, his left upper limb demonstrates flexing and the right upper limb demonstrates localising. What is his GCS?

A. 6
B. 7
C. 8
D. 9
E. 10

Q18:

A bodily fluid is being analysed for its composition and the following results are obtained: sodium 45mmol/l, potassium 5mmol/l, chloride 58mmol/l, bicarbonate 0mol/l and a pH of 5.2. Which body fluid is being analysed?

A. Saliva
B. Gastric juice
C. Bile
D. Sweat
E. Cerebrospinal fluid

Q19:

What is the respiratory compliance of a system if the chest wall compliance is $200mlcmH_2O^{-1}$ and the lung compliance is $200mlcmH_2O^{-1}$?

    A. $40000mlcmH_2O^{-1}$
    B. $400mlcmH_2O^{-1}$
    C. $200mlcmH_2O^{-1}$
    D. $100mlcmH_2O^{-1}$
    E. $1mlcmH_2O^{-1}$

Q20:

A patient is undergoing laparoscopic shoulder decompression surgery in the deck chair position. During the procedure, their end tidal carbon dioxide measurement slowly decreases and they develop sudden onset of cardiac instability, which progresses to cardiac arrest. What is the underlying aetiology?

    A. Venous air embolism
    B. Disconnection of patient from ventilator
    C. Massive haemothorax
    D. Tension pneumothorax
    E. Anaphylaxis

Q21:

Which of the following is not a physiological change of the respiratory system in pregnancy?

A. Tidal volume increases by 45%
B. Minute ventilation increases by 50%
C. Alveolar ventilation increases by 70%
D. Dead space increases by 45%
E. Expiratory reserve volume increases by 25%

Q22:

An intravenous anaesthetic agent has been developed with a molecular weight of 342. It is 50% protein bound and undergoes ester hydrolysis creating inactive metabolites that are 90% excreted in the urine. It is stored at room temperature in either propylene glycol or a lipid emulsion, giving it a pH of 8.1. It is contraindicated in porphyria. Which of the following statements is true?

A. Its molecular weight is less than sodium thiopental, propofol and ketamine
B. It is more protein bound than sodium thiopental and propofol
C. The molecule is more acidic than sodium thiopental in solution
D. Like propofol, it is contraindicated in porphyria
E. It is stored in a similar fashion to sodium thiopental

Q23:

You are using a circle system with a soda lime canister within the circle for a patient. If the patient produces 3 moles of carbon dioxide, how many moles of calcium carbonate will be produced?

    A. 0 moles
    B. 1 mole
    C. 2 moles
    D. 3 moles
    E. 4 moles

Q24:

A patient is undergoing spirometry and you ask them to maximally exhale after the end of expiration of a normal tidal volume. What volume will be measured?

    A. Inspiratory reserve volume
    B. Expiratory reserve volume
    C. Vital capacity
    D. Functional residual capacity
    E. Residual volume

Q25:

You are examining the contractile unit of myocytes and identify the Z line. Which is the correct definition of a Z line?

    A. The junction between neighbouring actin filaments that forms the border between sarcomeres
    B. The middle zone of the sarcomere
    C. The band encompassing the entire length of the myosin molecule
    D. The width of actin not overlapped by myosin
    E. The area where actin and myosin filaments overlap

Q26:

A circuit has two capacitors in parallel. Capacitor 1 has a capacitance of 20 farads and capacitor 2 has a capacitance of 10 farads. What is the total energy stored if a voltage of 10 volts is applied?

    A. 20 Joules
    B. 40 Joules
    C. 100 Joules
    D. 1500 Joules
    E. 2000 Joules

Q27:

Two separate inductors are wound around separate pieces of iron and placed in close proximity, so that a current is induced between the coils via a coupling effect of the magnetic fields. If coil 1 has 20 coils and an alternating current voltage of 100 volts and the second coil has 10 coils, what is the voltage in the second coil?

    A. 2 volts
    B. 20 volts
    C. 50 volts
    D. 130 volts
    E. 200 volts

Q28:

An 11 year old child weighing 30kg is scheduled to undergo emergency femoral fracture repair and you have been asked to prescribe a fluid bolus and a maintenance fluid regime. Which regime is most appropriate for the child?
    A. Fluid maintenance of 70mlhr^{-1} and a fluid bolus of 600ml
    B. Fluid maintenance of 110mlhr^{-1} and a fluid bolus of 600ml
    C. Fluid maintenance of 70mlhr^{-1} and a fluid bolus of 110ml
    D. Fluid maintenance of 110mlhr^{-1} and a fluid bolus of 110ml
    E. Fluid maintenance of 150mlhr^{-1} and a fluid bolus of 600ml

Q29:

Which of the following statements regarding the diaphragm is incorrect?

A. The inferior vena cava and right phrenic nerve traverse the diaphragm at T8.
B. The oesophagus and azygous vein traverse the diaphragm at T10
C. The aorta and thoracic duct traverse the diaphragm at T12
D. It contains three arcuate ligaments referred to as medial, lateral and median
E. The left crura is derived from the 1st and 2nd lumbar vertebra bodies and the right crura is derived from the 1st, 2nd and 3rd vertebral bodies

Q30:

You are dissecting the upper limb of a human specimen, which of the following statements is false regarding the muscles innervated by the median nerve?

A. The median nerve gives motor innervation to palmaris longus
B. The median nerve gives motor innervation to pronator teres
C. The median nerve gives motor innervation to flexor digitorum superficialis
D. The median nerve gives motor innervation to three thenar muscles
E. The median nerve gives motor innervation to the medial two lumbricals

Answers to Paper 1

Q1: D

This is a comparison of the chemical properties of inhalation anaesthetic agents and the only true statement is that the molecular weight is the same as isoflurane. It is important to be able to know the key values regarding inhalational agents and how this influences their clinical properties. In this question, the anaesthetic gas being described is enflurane.

Q2: A

The Nernst equation is concerned with how one ion affects the electrical potential of a cell, whereas, the Goldman equation takes into account numerous ions. The van't Hoff equation is concerned with the osmotic pressure exerted by a solution and the Gibbs-Donnan effect explains the movement of ions based on concentration and electrical potential. Stewart's strong ion theory is a way of explaining how dissociation of ionic compounds can effect the pH of a solution.

Q3: C

This is the classical presentation of organophosphate poisoning. Neostigmine, ecothiopate and pyridostigmine work in the same manner as industrial organophosphates and will make the situation worse. There is no role for intralipid in the management of organophosphate toxicity. Pralidoxime is meant to regenerate the toxin bound acetylcholinesterase. In the interim, atropine will be required to counter the effects of the organophosphate toxicity.

Q4: B

The Joint British Diabetes Societies for Inpatient Care (JBDS-IP) guideline for patients undergoing surgery in the United Kingdom was published in March 2016. In this situation they would recommend, as first line, prescribing 5% glucose with 0.45% saline and 0.15% potassium, though they acknowledge that this may not be freely available.

Q5: C
Whilst noradrenaline binds to alpha receptors and does not have beta adrenergic activity it has no bioavailability when given orally. Reserpine and methyl dopa are anti-hypertensives and the action of vasopressin is mediated by the stimulation of V_1 receptors. Midodrine has a high oral bioavailability and is a prodrug that can be used to treat orthostatic hypotension.

Q6: D
Heparin upregulates the activity of antithrombin III by a factor of 1000. Therefore, if no antithrombin is present the heparin will fail to work as an anticoagulant. This can occur in patients who have had prolonged courses of heparin therapy. Fresh frozen plasma contains antithrombin III which will enable the heparin to increase the APTT ratio for this patient.

Q7: A
The high central venous pressure and pulmonary capillary wedge pressure (PCWP) are highly suggestive of biventricular failure and the severe hypoxia demonstrates that the respiratory system is compromised. Traditionally ARDS requires normal PCWP and there is nothing to suggest the development of cardiac tamponade. Pneumonia and anaphylaxis should not increase PCWP, therefore pulmonary oedema is the most likely diagnosis.

Q8: A
Bone cement implantation syndrome and fat embolism should present intraoperatively during the cementing and nailing procedure. Anaphylaxis causes erythema and should be related to some administered agent. Pulmonary embolism would be unusual in such a

compromised patient who is not hypoxic. This procedure is notorious for blood loss and with this clinical picture, haemorrhagic hypovolaemia should be suspected as the most likely cause.

Q9: D

The "rule of nines" can be applied to an adult burns patient. In this scenario each leg would be 18%, the front of the abdomen and thorax another 18% and 1% for the genital area. This gives a total of 55%.

Q10: B

It is important to note that the epidural top-up did not contain adrenaline and the patient's weight means that the maximum safe dose would be 180mg (i.e. 3mg/kg without adrenaline). However, the patient received 400mg and presented with central neurology followed by cardiac collapse which would suggest local anaesthetic toxicity. A total spinal would have caused cardiac instability, followed by neurological features as it worked its way up to the brain. Anaphylaxis should not cause seizures and eclampsia should not cause bradycardia. A subdural catheter should cause a patchy block and a disproportionate motor weakness.

Q11: B

This clinical situation is describing a complete cord transection and you need to assess the level which is compromised. C2 would involve the muscles of respiration (including the phrenic nerve), so the patient would either be dead or require immediate ventilation. Below T6 he could respond to the loss of sympathetic tone in the legs by mounting a tachycardia but because he has a relative bradycardia and hypotension (with persevered breathing), the cord lesion must have stopped his cardiac sympathetic fibres. Hence B is the correct answer.

Q12: B

Kurtosis refers to the skewness of the normal distribution graph. A positive kurtosis means the normal distribution is shifted to the left whereas a negative kurtosis shifts to the right. When a positive kurtosis occurs, the mean is higher than the median which is greater than the mode.

Q13: C

Patients with myasthenia gravis have relative resistance to suxamethonium and neuromuscular blockade is prolonged by hypokalaemia and hypocalcaemia. Fentanyl does not affect neuromuscular recovery. Gentamicin prolongs the recovery for myasthenia gravis patients, as do lithium and calcium channel blockers.

Q14: E

Malignant hypertension is a serious condition which can cause all the condition listed. However, the patient is asymptomatic which makes B, C and D unlikely and A would require a profound reduction in eGFR, when he should be improving. More likely, is the fact that he has metabolised the sodium nitroprusside and developed cyanide toxicity as an unfortunate by product.

Q15: E

Canon A waves appear when the right atrium tries to contract against a closed tricuspid valve. This occurs when there is a dis-coordination between atrial and ventricular activity. Therefore, D and E are the possibilities. However, he has a tachycardia and not a bradycardia, therefore the answer is E.

Q16: A

Antipyrine can be used to estimate total body water, whereas radio-labelled sodium, mannitol and chloride give you the extracellular fluid. Radio-labelled albumin gives you the plasma volume.

Q17: D

When assessing a GCS in a patient you should always take the highest score as their GCS. In this scenario eyes score 2, verbal score is 2 and his best motor score is 5 (localising to pain). Therefore the total score is 9 out of 15.

Q18: D

Gastric juice is acidic with a pH of 3 and so can be excluded. Cerebrospinal fluid and bile have a similar sodium concentration to plasma at around 145mmol/l, so are incorrect. Saliva is more acidic than sweat with a higher potassium content, therefore the answer is sweat.

Q19: D

1/Respiratory compliance is equal to (1/chest wall compliance) + (1/ lung compliance), in a similar fashion to resistors in parallel. In this example it would be 1/200 + 1/200 which equals 2/200 which is simplified to 1/100. Therefore, respiratory compliance is 100ml/ cmH_2O.

Q20: A

All of the options listed can occur during shoulder surgery in the deck chair position. Disconnection from the ventilator should cause immediate cessation of the end tidal carbon dioxide measurement. Massive haemothorax, anaphylaxis and tension pneumothorax will reduce the end tidal carbon dioxide in extremis but the cardiac instability should occur first. This is a classical example of venous air embolism which can occur in any procedure requiring the deck chair position such as certain orthopaedic, neurosurgical and ENT procedures.

Q21: E

During pregnancy the tidal volume increases and as a result the alveolar ventilation increases. Due to the uterus increasing in size, the diaphragm is raised and as a result the expiratory reserve volume and functional residual capacity reduce.

Q22: C

The intravenous agent being described is etomidate. It is a large molecule that is less protein bound than sodium thiopental (80%) and propofol (98%). It has a pH of 8.1 in solution compared to sodium thiopental which is more alkaline at 10.5. Etomidate is contraindicated in porphyria whereas propofol is safe. Etomidate is stored as a liquid emulsion or in propylene glycol whereas sodium thiopental is stored as a powder in an inert gas.

Q23: D

The balanced chemical reaction for soda lime and CO_2 is as follows:

Step 1: $CO_2 + H_2O > H_2CO_3$

Step 2: $2NaOH + H_2CO_3 > Na_2CO_3 + 2H_2O + heat$

Step 3: $Na_2CO_3 + Ca(OH)_2 > CaCO_3 + 2NaOH + heat$

It is important to note the ratio of CO_2 entering at step 1 and the amount of calcium carbonate ($CaCO_3$) being produced is 1:1. Therefore, if 3 moles of carbon dioxide are added to the chemical reaction, 3 moles of calcium carbonate will be produced.

Q24: B

- Inspiratory reserve volume (IRV) is the volume of gas that can be further inhaled after a normal tidal breath until total lung capacity is reached.
- Expiratory reserve volume (ERV) is the functional residual capacity minus the residual volume and is the maximum amount of gas exhaled after a normal tidal volume.
- Residual volume is the volume of gas in the lung at the end of maximal exhalation.

- Functional residual capacity is the volume of gas in the lungs at the end of a normal tidal volume breath.
- Vital capacity is the sum of IRV + ERV + tidal volume.

Q25: A

The sarcomere is the contractile unit of the myocyte which contains interlocking actin and myosin filaments. The Z line occurs where the actin molecules join together perpendicular to the direction of the filament and is considered the border of the sarcomere.

Q26: D

The total capacitance of the circuit for capacitors in parallel is additive. Therefore, the total capacitance is 30 farads. The total energy stored can be found by the equation $1/2CV^2$. Placing the numbers into the equation you get the answer of 1500 joules.

For this question:

Total capacitance of circuit = 20 + 10 = 30 farads

Total stored energy = $1/2 \times 30 \times 10^2 = 1500$ Joules

Q27: C

This question is describing a step down transformer. Transformer 1 consisted of 20 coils with a voltage of 100v and transformer 2 has 10 coils with an unknown voltage.

The equation is:
Voltage at transformer 2 = voltage of transformer 1 x (n° of coils on 2/n° of coils on 1)

This works out to 50 volts as: 100 x (10/20) equals 50.

Q28: A

Maintenance fluid per hour for a child is calculated as 4ml/kg for the first 10kg of a child's weight, then 2ml/kg for the child's weight between 10-20kg and finally a further 1ml/kg for each subsequent kg above 20kg. A fluid bolus is 20ml/kg.

In this example a child weighing 30kg needs: (4 x10) + (2x10) + (1 x10) which equals 70mlhr^{-1} as maintenance and 600ml of fluid as a bolus (20 x 30).

Q29: B

All the statements about the diaphragm are correct except B. This is because the azygous vein travels with the aorta through the diaphragm at the level of T12.

Q30: E

The median nerve gives motor innervation to the lateral two lumbricals not the medial lumbricals.

Paper 2

Q1:

A patient presents to accident and emergency with bradycardia at 40 bpm and symptomatic heart failure. Atropine is administered with a satisfactory response. Which of the following features would not increase the patient's risk of asystole?

  A. Recent asystole
  B. Mobitz type II AV block
  C. Complete heart block with a broad QRS
  D. Ventricular pause of more than 3 seconds
  E. Patient currently on diltiazem

Q2:

A 4 year old child presents to accident and emergency in ventricular tachycardia without a pulse. Cardio-pulmonary resuscitation is started and the decision is made to defibrillate. Which is the appropriate energy level?

  A. 4 Joules
  B. 16 Joules
  C. 60 Joules
  D. 200 Joules
  E. 360 Joules

Q3:

A 45 year old patient undergoes elective varicose vein surgery in the prone position. He is intubated with propofol, rocuronium and fentanyl and then positioned without incident. 5 minutes later he develops a peak airway pressure of $40cmH_2O$ and SpO_2 reads 90%. He has a heart rate of 80bpm and a blood pressure of 100/40mmHg. What is the most likely underlying pathology?

A. One lung ventilation
B. Anaphylaxis
C. Incomplete neuromuscular blockade
D. Expected parameters for a patient in prone position
E. Opiate induced chest rigidity

Q4:

A patient is admitted through accident and emergency with a self inflicted stab wound to his groin. He has a heart rate of 110 bpm, blood pressure 110/90mmHg, respiratory rate of 20 breaths per minute and is mildly anxious. What is the likely blood loss?

A. Less than 750ml
B. 750-1500ml
C. 1500-2000ml
D. 2000-2500ml
E. More than 2500ml

Q5:

A patient presents to accident and emergency with a ruptured abdominal aortic aneurysm. He has developed hypovolaemic haemorrhagic shock and is booked for theatre. The patient's medication include dabigatran for atrial fibrillation. What is the optimal method to reverse the dabigatran?

A) Intravenous vitamin K
B) Fresh frozen plasma
C) Cryoprecipitate
D) Idarucizumab
E) Protamine

Q6:

Which of the following are possible features of the administration of morphine?

A. Increased release of ACTH
B. Increased prolactin release
C. Increased secretion of ADH
D. Stimulation of Edinger-Westphal nucleus resulting in the optic nerve causing pupil constriction
E. Decreased pressure in the biliary tree due to sphincter of Oddi spasm

Q7:

A 55 year old gentleman undergoes laparoscopic surgery for small bowel obstruction. He presented with a two week history of diarrhoea followed by nausea, vomiting and then an inability to pass flatus or stool. During the operation he develops acute peak airway pressure of $40cmH_20$, a heart rate increase to 130bpm and a flushed appearance. What is the most appropriate management?

A. Administer octreotide
B. Administer aminophylline
C. Administer adrenaline
D. Administer hydrocortisone
E. Administer rocuronium

Q8:

Which of the following is not a cause of hypercalcaemia?

A. Multiple endocrine neoplasia type I
B. Sarcoidosis
C. Parathyroid adenoma
D. Peutz-Jeghers syndrome
E. Tuberculosis

Q9:

A 76 year old male is intubated on intensive care with suspected meningitis. The cerebrospinal fluid sample has grown a gram positive organism that forms cocci. What is the likely pathogen?

    A. Streptococcus pneumoniae
    B. Neisseria meningitidis
    C. Haemophilus influenza
    D. Listeria monocytogenes
    E. Tuberculosis

Q10:

Which of the following statements is false regarding the male inguinal canal?

    A. It is bordered by inguinal ligament inferiorly
    B. It is bordered by the aponeurosis of the external oblique anteriorly
    C. It is bordered by the conjoint tendon and fascia transervsalis posteriorly
    D. The ilioinguinal and hypogastric nerve traverse the canal
    E. The spermatic cord contains the vas deferent, pampiniform plexus and genital branch of the genitofemoral nerve

Q11:

The following are accurate statements regarding the anatomical borders of the antecubital fossa with the exception of:

A. It is bordered inferomedially by pronator teres
B. It is bordered inferolaterally by brachioradialis
C. It is bordered superiorly by a line joining the humeral epicondyles
D. Its roof is the deep fascia reinforced by bicipital aponeurosis
E. Its floor is flexor digitorum profundus

Q12:

A constant flow rate of liquid is applied to a length of tubing. Point A of the tubing has twice the cross sectional area of point B of the tubing. Which of the following statements is false?

A. The velocity of the fluid is less at point A than point B
B. The pressure at point B is greater than that at point A
C. The kinetic and potential energy of the system are linked to a constant if no energy is added or taken away
D. The liquid has to be incompressible to determine relationships between pressure and flow in the system
E. Bernoulli's equation describes how kinetic and potential energy changes in this system

Q13:

A simple electric circuit is created with a single resistor with a resistance of 20 ohms. When a current of 10 amps is applied to the circuit what will the power of the circuit become?

A. 2 watts
B. 30 watts
C. 200 watts
D. 2000 watts
E. 4000 watts

Q14:

Methoxyflurane is administered via an inhalation patient-triggered device for a patient with a fractured distal radius. Later that day they patient is taken to theatre for definitive surgical management. Which of the following drugs should be avoided?

A. Desflurane
B. Enflurane
C. Halothane
D. Isoflurane
E. Sevoflurane

Q15:

A 35 year old male presents to emergency services with life threatening asthma. He receives oxygen, salbutamol and ipratropium nebulisers, magnesium sulphate and hydrocortisone. Which of the following is not a feature of life threatening asthma?

A. Peak expiratory flow rate of less than 33% of predicted
B. Pulse oximetry of less than 92%
C. Respiratory rate of more than 24 breaths per minute
D. Arrhythmia
E. $PaCO_2$ of 4.6-6kPa

Q16:

You are dissecting the human larynx on a cadaver. Which of the following intrinsic muscles of the larynx is not supplied by the recurrent laryngeal nerve?

A. Cricothyroid
B. Posterior crico-arytenoid
C. Lateral crico-arytenoid
D. Thyroarytenoid
E. Vocalis

Q17:

An experiment is undertaken to see how the oxygen-haemoglobin dissociation curve is changed by altering different variables. The control shows a p50 value occurring at a partial pressure of 3.5kPa of oxygen tension. When a particular variable is altered, the p50 value occurs at 4kPa. Which of the following variables could account for the change in the p50 value?

    A. Decreasing the amount of 2,3-diphosphoglycerate
    B. Increasing the temperature
    C. Decreased partial pressure of carbon dioxide
    D. Increased pH
    E. Creation of methaemoglobin

Q18:

A 24 year old patient undergoes diagnostic laparoscopic surgery for suspected endometriosis. Which of the following physiological complications would not be expected to occur?

    A. Decrease in cardiac output
    B. Increase in renal blood flow
    C. Decrease in preload
    D. Increase in intracranial pressure
    E. Decrease in splanchnic blood flow

Q19:

An awake interscalene block is being performed for laparoscopic shoulder surgery. During the procedure the patient develops an alteration in their mental status and progresses to a loss of consciousness. At the same time they develop cardiovascular collapse with hypotension and sinus bradycardia with variable conduction blocks. What is the cause of the patient's deterioration?

A. Tension pneumothorax
B. Anaphylaxis
C. Total spinal
D. Local anaesthetic toxicity
E. Massive haemothorax

Q20:

A patient undergoes a laparotomy for small bowel adhesions. He is maintained on sevoflurane intraoperatively and his medications includes propranolol, diltiazem, isosorbide mononitrate and salbutamol as needed. Which of the following medications could potentiate hypoxic pulmonary vasoconstriction under anaesthesia?

A. Sevoflurane
B. Isosorbide mononitrate
C. Propranolol
D. Diltiazem
E. Salbutamol

Q21:

A 4 year old child presents to accident and emergency with an exacerbation of asthma. Salbutamol is administered via inhaler and then by nebuliser and prednisolone is given orally. Which of the following is not a feature of life threatening asthma in this child?

A. Cyanosis
B. Poor respiratory effort
C. Hypotension
D. Too breathless to talk
E. Silent chest

Q22:

A patient is maintained on an inhalation anaesthetic vapour with the following properties: molecular weight of 74, boiling point of 35°C, saturated vapour pressure of 7.8kPa, blood gas co-efficient 12.1 and an oil gas co-efficient of 65. It is 15% metabolised in the body to carbon dioxide and water. Which anaesthetic gas is being described?

A. Enflurane
B. Ether
C. Halothane
D. Methoxyflurane
E. Xenon

Q23:

A 35 year old man is intubated on intensive care due to symptomatic acute hyponatraemia. He is considered euvolaemic and his urine osmolality is greater than 100mOsmkg^{-1} with plasma hypo-osmolality. What is a possible diagnosis with this clinical presentation?

A. Syndrome of inappropriate anti-diuretic hormone secretion (SIADH)
B. Cerebral salt wasting syndrome
C. Nephrotic syndrome
D. Diuretic use
E. Pancreatitis

Q24:

The Joule is a measure of the amount of work done. 1 joule is equivalent to which of the following conversions?

A. 1 Kg.m^2.s^{-2}
B. 1 W (watt)
C. 1kW (kilowatt)
D. 1eV (electron volt)
E. 1 calorie

Q25:

A 55 year old man with myasthenia gravis undergoes a repair of umbilical hernia under general anaesthesia. After the procedure he is intubated and requires a prolonged stay on intensive care. Which of the following is not a risk factor for requiring prolonged ventilation post-operatively in a patient with myasthenia gravis?

A. Presence of disease for more than 6 years
B. Co-existing respiratory disease
C. Vital capacity of less than 2.9 litres
D. Taking more than 750mg pyridostigmine daily
E. Peak expiratory flow rate less than 480 litres per minute

Q26:

A 24 year old man presents to accident and emergency with acute onset of blurred vision, difficulty swallowing and bilateral facial weakness. He also complains of abdominal cramps. Over the course of 24 hours he progresses to respiratory failure requiring ventilation. He has preserved sensation throughout. What is the likely diagnosis?

A. Guillian-Barre syndrome
B. Botulism
C. Myasthenia gravis
D. Stroke
E. Chronic inflammatory demyelinating polyneuropathy

Q27:

An infant presents to the paediatric emergency services with dehydration caused by vomiting and diarrhoea. The child has a sunken anterior fontanelle, decreased skin turgor, dry mucus membranes with sunken eyes and an increased respiratory and pulse rate. The child is catheterised and has made less than 1ml/kg of urine in the last hour. How much fluid has the child lost as a percentage of body weight?

A. 5%
B. 10%
C. 15%
D. 20%
E. 30%

Q28:

A 4 month old child presents to paediatric services with severe dehydration and history of projectile vomiting. Pyloric stenosis is suspected. Which of the following biochemical phenomena would you not expect to find in this child?

A. Hypernatraemia
B. Hypokalaemia
C. Hypochloraemia
D. Low urinary sodium concentration
E. Plasma alkalosis

Q29:

A new diuretic has been approved for the management of hypertension. Its mechanism of action is to block the potassium/sodium/chloride symporter on the apical surface of the thick ascending limb of the loop of Henle, which thereby inhibits the kidneys countercurrent multiplication process. Which class of diuretics does the drug belong to?

    A. Osmotic diuretics
    B. Loop diuretics
    C. Thiazide diuretics
    D. Carbonic anhydrase diuretics
    E. Potassium sparing diuretics

Q30:

You are measuring the lung volume of a patient due to undergo elective oesophagectomy. Which of the following equations would give an equal volume to the functional residual capacity?

    A. Residual volume plus expiratory reserve volume
    B. Total lung capacity minus vital capacity
    C. Vital capacity minus tidal volume
    D. Total lung capacity minus residual volume
    E. Expiratory reserve volume plus inspiratory reserve volume

Answers to Paper 2

Q1: E
The Advanced Life Support algorithm lists risks factors for developing asystole in a bradycardic patient. They include all of the list, with the exception of taking diltiazem.

Q2: C
The Paediatric Advanced Life Support algorithm states that an energy of 4 joules per kilogram should be used to defibrillate a child. At the age of 4 the child should weigh 16Kg using the equation: weight = (age + 4) x 2. Therefore, 60 Joules would be the nearest most appropriate energy level. As the child has a pulseless ventricular tachycardia a defibrillation attempt is warranted.

Q3: A
Prone positioning has many potentially serious complications. In this case, the cause is unlikely to be incomplete neuromuscular blockade, as intubation has just occurred with a moderately long acting relaxant. He is cardiovascularly stable with no rash, making anaphylaxis unlikely. Whilst chest wall rigidity can occur with opiates, this usually occurs at much higher doses than those used in varicose vein surgery. This degree of hypoxia and poor compliance is not expected in the prone position. A common complication of prone surgery is one lung ventilation, as the tube can advance during the positioning, ultimately leading to hypoxia and high airway pressures. Likewise, accidental extubation has also been described with this position.

Q4: B
Haemorrhage shock can be classified as grade I, II, III or IV. These grades correspond, respectively, to blood losses of up to 750ml (up to 15%), 750-1500ml (15-30%), 1500-2000ml (30-40%) or greater

than 2000ml (40%). Dependant on the degree of shock the clinical presentation alters and in this instance 750-1500ml of blood loss would be expected.

Q5: D

Dabigatran is a direct thrombin inhibitor that is licensed for numerous conditions. Until recently it had no reliable antidote and it has made the management of the actively bleeding patient difficult. Recently, a new monoclonal antibody has been licensed which immediately reverses the effects of dabigatran. For this patient vitamin K would have no effect, nor would cryoprecipitate and protamine would only reverse heparin. In the past, FFP was used to try and improve the clotting activity of a patient on dabigatran, but was unreliable.

Q6: C

Opiates reduce the secretion of all pituitary hormones except ADH. Whilst it is true that opiates cause pupillary construction via stimulation of the Edinger-Westphal nucleus, it is incorrect that the optic nerve carries the motor nerve fibres (it is the occulomotor nerve). Spasm of the sphincter of Oddi will increase biliary pressure.

Q7: A

This is the typical presentation of carcinoid syndrome. The patient is middle-aged and experiencing the bowel symptoms of excess serotonin. With the stress of surgery and the handling of the tumour around the appendix, a carcinoid crisis occurred with bronchospasm. The appropriate medication in this instance is octreotide.

Q8: D

Peutz-Jeghers syndrome is an autosomal dominant condition that causes hamartomatous polyps to form in the gastrointestinal tract and causes pigmentation of mucus membranes. It is not associated with hypercalcaemia, unlike the other conditions.

Q9: A

Neisseria meningitidis and haemophilus are gram negative pathogens. Listeria is gram positive but forms rods not cocci. Tuberculosis does not retain any bacteriological stain due to the high lipid content of its cell wall (a Ziehl-Neelsen stain is instead used). Streptococcus is gram positive and forms cocci. All the pathogens can cause meningitis.

Q10: D

The iliohypogastric nerve does not traverse the inguinal canal, but is blocked as part of a field block for inguinal surgery.

Q11: E

The floor of the ante-cubital fossa is supinator laterally and brachialis medially.

Q12: B

The Bernoulli equation describes how a fall in kinetic energy results in a gain in potential energy and vice versa, on the provision that no energy is either added or taken away from the system (and the substance flowing is incompressible). Therefore, at a constriction, the flow increases (i.e. the kinetic energy) but the pressure subsequently falls (potential energy). Therefore, B is a false statement.

Q13: D

Power = current^2 x resistance
For this example: 10^2 x 20 = 2000
The unit of power is the watt which is equivalent to joules per second.

Q14: E

Methoxyflurane has been used in Australia for many years as a form of patient-triggered analgesia in emergency situations. The device has a charcoal canister to prevent people near the patient being exposed to anaesthetic gas. The risk of methoxyflurane in combination with sevoflurane is renal dysfunction due to an accumulation of fluoride ions.

Q15: C
The British Thoracic Society has guidelines regarding the diagnosis and management of stable and unstable asthma in adults and children. In emergency situations it can be classified as near fatal, life threatening, severe or moderate. In this example, a respiratory rate of more than 24 breaths per minute is in the category of severe asthma, not life threatening asthma.

Q16: A
The recurrent laryngeal nerve supplies all the intrinsic muscles of the larynx except the cricothyroid muscle, which is supplied by the external branch of the superior laryngeal nerve.

Q17: B
This question is demonstrating a right shift in the oxygen-haemoglobin dissociation curve as the p50 value is occurring at a higher partial pressure. The only option that will shift the curve to the right is increasing the temperature, all the other options will shift the curve to the left.

Q18: B
Inflation of the abdominal cavity to cause a pneumoperitoneum reduces venous return, thereby reducing the preload to the heart and ultimately reducing the cardiac output. The pneumoperitoneum increases after load and in combination with reduced cardiac output, will reduce splanchnic and renal blood flow. The head down position and increased abdominal pressure will increase intra-cranial pressure.

Q19: D

All of the listed complications can occur with an inter-scalene blockade. Anaphylaxis, massive haemothorax and tension pneumothorax would usually result in tachycardia. Total spinal would result in loss of consciousness but the addition of the cardiovascular effects means that local anaesthetic toxicity is the most likely option.

Q20: C
Medications and biological chemicals that potentiate hypoxic pulmonary vasoconstriction (HPV) are favourite questions in anaesthetic examinations. In this example propranolol would have potentiated HPV, as the other agents would reduce the HPV drive.

Q21: D
The British Thoracic Society has guidelines regarding the diagnosis and management of stable and unstable asthma in adults and children. In this example, being too breathless to talk is a sign of acute severe asthma whereas the others are features of life threatening asthma.

Q22: B
These are the properties of ether. It is the only anaesthetic agent that is metabolised to water and carbon dioxide.

Q23: A
The syndrome of inappropriate ADH secretion (SIADH) has many causes and is characterised by:
- euvolaemia
- hypotonia
- hyponatraemia
- inappropriately high urinary osmolality and urine sodium concentration

Cerebral salt wasting syndrome, diuretic use and pancreatitis produce a hypovolaemic hyponatraemia and nephrotic syndrome produces a hypervolaemic state.

The mainstay of treatment for SIADH is fluid restriction to around 1000ml per day and the slow correction of sodium by 1.5mmol/l per day. Other potential treatments include hypertonic saline (which should only be used with extreme caution in severe hyponatraemic and symptomatic patients), furosemide and other diuretics, demeclocycline (which inhibits the renal response to ADH) and ADH receptor antagonists such as conivaptan.

Q24: A
A watt is a joule per second, therefore a kilowatt and watt are incorrect. Calories and electronvolts are derived units of energy similar to a joule but are not of equal magnitude (1 calorie equals 4.184 joules and 1 electronvolt equals 1.6×10^{-19} joules). Therefore the answer is $1\ Kg.m^2.s^{-2}$.

Q25: E
Features A, B, C and D are well described as increasing the need for prolonged ventilation in a patient with myasthenia gravis. The peak expiratory flow rate in this example is not particularly poor and is not associated with the prognosis regarding the need for post-operative ventilation.

Q26: B
Botulism toxicity traditionally presents with a sore throat, drooling and a descending motor weakness that can effect the cranial nerves. Gillian-Barre syndrome (excluding Miller Fisher syndrome) and chronic inflammatory demyelinating polyneuropathy present with an ascending motor paralysis with spared sensation. It would be unlikely to be a stroke syndrome as a bilateral facial weakness would involve both hemispheres.

Q27: B
Dehydration of a child can be divided into mild, moderate and severe depending on whether they have lost up to 5, 5-10 or more than 15%

of their body weight in fluid. The clinical picture described would be of a child that has lost 5-10% of their body weight in fluid.

Q28: A

Pyloric stenosis presents with metabolic alkalosis with hypochloraemia, hypokalaemia and potentially hyponatraemia. The child has losses from the stomach in the form of fluid, acid and potassium. The kidney attempts to preserve chloride and sodium at the expense of bicarbonate and potassium. A useful marker of adequate fluid resuscitation is when the urinary chloride level returns to normal.

Q29: B

Inhibition of the potassium/sodium/chloride symporter is the mechanism of action of loop diuretics on the thick ascending loop of Henle.

Q30: A

Functional residual capacity is the volume of gas in the lungs at the end of a normal tidal volume. As such the volume remaining in the lung at this point is the combination of the expiratory reserve volume and residual volume.

Paper 3

Q1:

You are investigating factors that affect pulmonary vascular resistance. Which of the following will not increase pulmonary vascular resistance in a human subject?

    A. Thromboxane A2
    B. Acetylcholine
    C. Serotonin
    D. Histamine
    E. Carbon dioxide

Q2:

Carbon dioxide is carried in the blood as carb-amino compounds, bicarbonate and in its dissolved form. As the carbon dioxide travels from the arterial to venous phase how does the percentage transport of carbon dioxide alter?

    A. More is dissolved, more is in the form of bicarbonate and less is in the carb-amino compound form
    B. Less is dissolved, less in carb-amino compound form and more in bicarbonate form
    C. More is dissolved, more in carb-amino compound form and less in bicarbonate
    D. More in bicarbonate form, more in carb-amino compound form and less in dissolved form
    E. More in dissolved form, less in carb-amino compound form and less in bicarbonate form

Q3:

In the human kidney, which of the following does not increase afferent arteriole pressure?

A. Angiotensin II
B. Adrenaline
C. Vasopressin
D. Prostaglandins
E. Endothelin

Q4:

Foetal haemoglobin differs from adult haemoglobin in all of the following ways except?

A. It consists of two alpha and two gamma chains
B. It binds 2,3-diphophoglyceric acid more avidly than adult haemoglobin
C. It results in a left shift of the oxygen-haemoglobin dissociation curve
D. It has a p50 value of 2.4kPa
E. Its difference in structure to adult haemoglobin favours maternal offloading of oxygen to foetal haemoglobin

Q5:

The Overton-Meyer hypothesis links the oil gas partition co-efficient to the minimum alveolar concentration (MAC) of an agent. Which of the following statements regarding this relationship is true?

A. To form a linear relationship, both MAC and oil gas partition co-efficients need a logarithmic transformation
B. To form a linear relationship, the MAC requires logarithmic transformation
C. To form a linear relationship, the oil gas partition co-efficient requires logarithmic transformation
D. To form a linear relationship, neither factor needs representing in logarithmic form
E. Logarithmic transformation of MAC and oil gas co-efficient results in an exponential curve

Q6:

A 93 year old lady is scheduled to undergo fixation of a fractured neck of femur and you review her on the ward. Which of the following is not an acceptable reason for postponing surgery?

A. Haemoglobin less than 10g/dl
B. Plasma sodium less than 120mmol/l
C. Chest infection with sepsis
D. Reversible coagulopathy
E. Acute left ventricular failure

Q7:

You perform a very challenging epidural for a patient in labour for analgesia. She has a BMI of 55kgm⁻², borderline platelet count, extreme needle phobia and has had previous spinal surgery. On performing the epidural you get clear fluid from the tuohy needle that is positive for glucose. Which of the following is the most appropriate management?

    A. Perform normal test dose
    B. Commence normal epidural infusion rate without a bolus
    C. Repeat the epidural process
    D. Label as a spinal catheter and treat as if a spinal catheter
    E. Use an opiate free epidural infusion

Q8:

You are investigating the cardiac output of a patient awaiting oesophagectomy and calculate the following values: arterial oxygen saturation of haemoglobin 100%, venous oxygen saturation of haemoglobin 75%, haemoglobin 10g/dl, arterial PaO_2 10kPa, venous PaO_2 6kPa and a heart rate 100 bpm with a stroke volume of 70ml. The patient is male, 60 years old, 1.75m tall and 70kg. Which of the following statements is false?

    A. The data is uninterpretable as we do not know the FiO_2 that the patient was on at the time of data collection
    B. His cardiac output can be calculated from this data
    C. His cardiac index can be calculated from this data
    D. His body mass index can be calculated from this data
    E. His body surface are can be calculated by the Du Bois formula

Q9:

A 24 year old presents to accident and emergency with a narrow complex tachyarrhythmia at 180bpm, which you suspect is a supra-ventricular tachycardia (SVT). He has a normal blood pressure, no chest pain, has not fainted and is not in pulmonary oedema. What is your first step in the management of this patient?

    A. Electrical cardioversion
    B. Adenosine 6mg
    C. Adenosine 12mg
    D. Verapamil 2.5-5mg
    E. Vagal manoeuvres

Q10:

A 32 year old patient with type II diabetes mellitus is due to undergo a total knee replacement under enhanced recovery on a morning list. Her current medication is novomix 30 twice daily. How should her insulin regime be managed on the day of surgery?

    A. Stop and place on a variable rate insulin infusion
    B. Half the morning dose of novomix 30 and leave the evening meal dose unchanged
    C. Half the morning dose and evening dose of novomix 30
    D. Continue current regime without change
    E. Convert to oral hypoglycaemic agents

Q11:

A 24 year old woman is involved in a road traffic accident and sustains an open bimalleolar ankle fracture. You review her analgesic requirements on the ward. Which of the following medications has the lowest number needed to treat (NNT) to reduce pain scores by 50%?

  A. Diclofenac 100mg
  B. Co-codamol (Codeine 60mg and Paracetamol 1g)
  C. Oxycodone immediate release 5mg and paracetamol 500mg
  D. Ibuprofen 800mg
  E. Tramadol 50mg

Q12:

A 35 year old gentleman with type II diabetes mellitus is started on a variable rate insulin infusion (VRII) regime as he is due to undergo major abdominal surgery and is not expected to eat and drink normally for 48 hours. Which of the following diabetes medications can he continue to take whilst on his VRII?

  A. Acarbose
  B. Metformin
  C. Pioglitazone
  D. DPP IV inhibitor (i.e. sitagliptin)
  E. GLP-1 analogue (i.e. exenatide)

Q13:

You are investigating the ratio of inertial forces to viscous forces within a fluid and derive the following data: density of liquid 100kgm^{-3}, flow velocity 100ms^{-1}, diameter 10mm and viscosity 5Nsm^{-2}. Which of the following statements is correct?

    A. Reynold's number is 20,000, therefore flow will be turbulent
    B. Reynold's number is 50, therefore flow will be laminar
    C. Reynold's number will be 200, therefore flow will be laminar
    D. Reynold's number will be 20,000, therefore flow will be laminar
    E. Reynold's number will be 50, therefore flow will be turbulent

Q14:

You are dissecting the orbit of the human eye and are interested in the nerves which traverse the superior orbital fissure. Which of the following nerves does not traverse the superior orbital fissure?

    A. Lacrimal nerve
    B. Frontal nerve
    C. Trochlear nerve
    D. Abducens nerve
    E. Optic nerve

Q15:

A 31 year old lady is requesting an epidural for analgesia in labour. She has a history of idiopathic thrombocytopenia and her current platelet count is 80×10^9/litre within the last 24 hours. How would you categorise her risk of complication?

A. Reduced risk
B. Normal risk
C. Increased risk
D. High risk
E. Very high risk

Q16:

A patient presents to the accident and emergency department after taking a staggered overdose of paracetamol. Which of the following is not included in the assessment of liver failure severity due to paracetamol?

A. Arterial pH
B. International normalised ratio (INR)
C. Serum creatinine
D. Degree of encephalopathy
E. Bilirubin

Q17:

A patient has a thoracic epidural sited to provide post operative analgesia after an elective abdominal aortic aneurysm repair. On the ward he is just able to flex his knees with free movement of the feet. How would you categorise his Brommage scale?

A. Grade 1
B. Grade 2
C. Grade 3
D. Grade 4
E. Unable to categorise as epidural infusion running

Q18:

A patient undergoes emergency surgery for a dental abscess which is causing respiratory distress. Prior to the anaesthetic he had a hoarse voice, drooling, inability to swallow and significant trismus. He was a grade III intubation. After the surgery he has no cuff leak when the cuff is deflated. What is the appropriate management for this patient after surgery?

A. Post-pone extubation and keep ventilated on the intensive care unit
B. Perform tracheostomy
C. Exchange tracheal tube for laryngeal mask airway
D. Extubate awake on remifentanil
E. Use an airway exchange catheter

Q19:

A 50kg female presents with 20% burns to the surface of her body. What would be the expected fluid maintenance rate per hour for the first 24 hour period?

    A. 30mlhr^{-1}
    B. 42mlhr^{-1}
    C. 70mlhr^{-1}
    D. 167mlhr^{-1}
    E. 200mlhr^{-1}

Q20:

Which of the following is not a renal adaptation encountered during pregnancy?

    A. Increased renal plasma flow
    B. Increased glomerular filtration rate
    C. Increased urinary volume
    D. Increased renal tubular reabsorption
    E. Increased creatinine clearance

Q21:

A 44 year old patient undergoes laparoscopic cholecystectomy and has his anaesthesia maintained with sevoflurane. During the surgery he develops a temperature of 41°C, end tidal carbon dioxide rise to 8kPa despite adequate ventilation and a heart rate of 160bpm. Which of the following is not a recommended treatment for the complications of this condition?

A. Treat hyperkalaemia with calcium chloride, glucose/insulin infusion and sodium bicarbonate
B. Treat arrhythmias with magnesium, amiodarone or metoprolol
C. Treat metabolic acidosis with hyperventilation, muscle relaxation with depolarising neuromuscular agent and sodium bicarbonate
D. Treat myoglobinaemia with mannitol, furosemide and sodium bicarbonate
E. Treat disseminated intravascular coagulopathy with fresh frozen plasma, platelets and cryoprecipitate

Q22:

An antiplatelet agent works by inhibiting the ADP receptor expressed on platelet cell membranes. It is administered as a prodrug and is activated in the liver by cytochrome p450 enzymes. Compared to similar drugs it has a longer duration of action and requires once daily administration. It rarely causes agranulocytosis and pancreatitis. Which drug is being described?

A. Clopidogrel
B. Ticagrelor
C. Aspirin
D. Fondaparinux
E. Tirofiban

Q23:

A patient undergoes fore foot surgery under general anaesthesia with an ankle block. When the patient wakes in recovery they complain of pain over the dorsal aspect of the foot. Which nerve has been inadequately blocked?

A. Superficial peroneal nerve
B. Deep peroneal nerve
C. Sural nerve
D. Tibial nerve
E. Saphenous nerve

Q24:

An anaesthetic breathing circuit fresh gas supply requires 2 to 3 times the minute ventilation of a spontaneously breathing patient to prevent rebreathing of carbon dioxide and approximately 70ml/kg/min with an intermittent positive pressure ventilation to maintain an arterial partial pressure of carbon dioxide of 5.3kPa. Which Mapleson circuit is being described?

    A. Mapleson A
    B. Mapleson B
    C. Mapleson C
    D. Mapleson D
    E. Mapleson E

Q25:

A sealed jar contains multiple gasses which when their partial pressures are added to together gives a total pressure inside the jar of 100kPa. Which gas law is being demonstrated by adding the partial pressures?

    A. Boyle's law
    B. Charles' law
    C. Dalton's Law
    D. Gay-Lussac's law
    E. Universal gas constant

Q26:

A patient undergoes a Bier's block for manipulation of a distal radial fracture with prilocaine. During the procedure it is noticed that they turn a dusky blue colour. What is the mechanism of action behind the observed phenomena?

A. The prilocaine in susceptible individuals causes red cell sickling

B. The iron oxidation state in haemoglobin is reduced by the prilocaine

C. The iron oxidation state in haemoglobin is oxidised by the prilocaine

D. The patient developed immune mediated histamine release

E. The Bier's block has caused phrenic nerve paralysis resulting in hypoventilation

Q27:

A drug exhibits tautomerism and has an ionised structure at pH of 4 and a non-ionised form when the pH is 7.4. The drug makes a seven membered ring structure in the non-ionised form. Which drug is being described?

A. Actracurium

B. Bupivocaine

C. Ketamine

D. Midazolam

E. Sodium thiopental

Q28:

You are investigating the laminar flow of liquids in tubing, which of the following options will increase flow rate the most?

    A. Doubling the radius of the tube
    B. Halving the radius of the tube
    C. Doubling the pressure gradient
    D. Halving the viscosity
    E. Doubling the length of the tube

Q29:

A 33 year old gentleman with acute intermittent porphyria undergoes emergency surgery for a pilonidal abscess under general anaesthesia. He is anaesthetised with sodium thiopental, suxamethonium, fentanyl and atracurium. Anaesthesia is maintained with nitrous oxide and enflurane. Which agent is the most likely to precipitate an acute porphyria crisis?

    A. Actracurium
    B. Fentanyl
    C. Nitrous oxide
    D. Sodium thiopental
    E. Suxamethonium

Q30:

An 18 year old is intubated and ventilated on intensive care after a traumatic brain injury. His investigations reveal a plasma sodium of 150mmol/l, a serum osmolality of 315mmol/kg and a low urine osmolality of 330 mmol/kg with an increased urinary output of 3500ml/day and relative hypovolaemia. What is the likely diagnosis?

A. Cerebral salt wasting syndrome
B. Diabetes insipidus
C. Excess sodium intake
D. Normal
E. Syndrome of inappropriate ADH secretion (SIADH)

Answers to Paper 3

Q1: B

Acetylcholine reduces pulmonary vascular resistance whereas all the other agents increase pulmonary vascular resistance.

Q2: C

In the venous circulation, the off loading of oxygen from haemoglobin allows the haemoglobin molecule to then combine with carbon dioxide forming a carb-amino compound (the Haldane effect). Carbon dioxide produced is freely able to dissolve in the plasma and so the amount of dissolved carbon dioxide increases. Ultimately the change observed in carbon dioxide transport between arterial and venous phases can be described as: more is dissolved (5% arterial and 10% venous), more in carb-amino compounds (5% arterial and 30% venous) and less in bicarbonate form (90% arterial and 60% venous).

Q3: D

Constriction at the afferent arteriole in the kidney is controlled by angiotensin II, adrenaline, endothelin, adenosine, vasopressin and prostaglandin blockade.

Q4: B

Foetal haemoglobin is left shifted on the oxygen-haemoglobin dissociation curve as it needs to extract oxygen from the maternal haemoglobin. Therefore, the p50 value of foetal haemoglobin is lowered so it does not utilise 2,3-dpg, otherwise it would move the curve inappropriately to the right. Foetal haemoglobin has a different protein structure to adult haemoglobin, with foetal haemoglobin having two alpha and two gamma subunits as opposed to the two alpha and two beta subunits of adult haemoglobin.

Q5: A

The Overton-Meyer hypothesis describes how the increasing oil gas partition co-efficient of an anaesthetic agent improves the potency of an inhalation agent. Potency in anaesthesia is described using a minimum alveolar concentration (MAC) concept (with more potent agents having a lower MAC value). This relationship is non-linear unless both MAC and the oil gas partition coefficient are transformed into logarithmic form.

Q6: A

The Association of Anaesthetists of Great Britain and Ireland (AAGBI) have produced a document regarding the care of patients with fractured neck of femurs. Options B, C, D and E are all appropriate reasons to delay surgery. They consider a haemoglobin concentration of less than 8g/dl to be an appropriate reason to delay surgery (not 10g/dl).

Q7: D

This is a challenging patient for technical, psychiatric and clinical reasons. From the clinical vignette it is highly likely that a dural tap has occurred and in clinical practice it would be important to follow the departmental policy. In this example, it would be extremely difficult to reattempt the epidural and there is no guarantee that it would be successful. Threading the catheter and either commencing the normal epidural infusion or giving the normal test dose risks the catastrophe of either a total spinal or profound hypotension resulting in foetal and maternal compromise. An opiate free solution will not alter how the infusion behaves and should not be considered. If the catheter is threaded and treated as a spinal catheter from the start then safe analgesia could be offered to the mother and it would be the preferred option. In this event it is vital that the anaesthetists administer top ups, that the catheter is labelled and no infusion is commenced.

Q8: A

The Fick principle requires a knowledge of the difference between arterial and venous blood oxygen content and its uptake, so does not require knowledge of the FiO_2. From the information provided in the question, we can calculate the delivery of oxygen to the tissues and the amount of oxygen used. As we are given the height and weight of the patient, we can calculate body surface with the Du Bois formula and body mass index. The combination of being able to calculate the cardiac output and body surface area enables us to calculate his cardiac index.

Q9: E

The patient does not have any of the Advanced Life Support features of compromise (i.e. chest pain, pulmonary oedema, syncope or hypotension), therefore cardioversion is currently not warranted. Whilst adenosine can be administered starting at 6mg and then increasing the dose, it would be wise to start with non-pharmacological treatments in the stable patient such as vagal manoeuvres. Given his age, carotid massage or valsalva should be safe. Verapamil is reserved for patients who are intolerant to adenosine who need pharmacological intervention.

Q10: B

The Joint British Diabetes Societies for Inpatient Care (JBDS-IP) guideline for patients undergoing surgery in the United Kingdom was published in March 2016. In this situation they would recommend halving the morning dose of novomix 30 and leaving the evening dose unchanged.

Q11: A

The Oxford Pain Group League Table of Analgesic Efficacy is an evidenced based review of different analgesics in terms of a number needed to treat (NNT) to reduce pain by 50%. Ibuprofen 800mg has a NNT of 1.6, diclofenac 100mg has a NNT of 1.9, co-codamol

(60mg/1g) has a NNT of 2.2, oxycodone immediate release 5mg and paracetamol 500mg have a NNT of 2.2 and tramadol 50mg has a NNT of 8.3. Therefore ibuprofen 800mg is the correct answer.

Q12: E

The Joint British Diabetes Societies for Inpatient Care (JBDS-IP) guideline for patients undergoing surgery in the United Kingdom was published in March 2016. In this situation they would recommend continuing his exenatide and not the other medications.

Q13: A

Reynold's number is calculated by multiplying the density, velocity and diameter of the tube and then dividing this number by the viscosity. In this example Reynold's number is 20,000. It is generally considered that values greater than 2000 will cause turbulent flow, hence the answer is A.

Q14: E

The optic nerve traverses the optic canal with the ophthalmic artery. The superior orbital fissure contains the lacrimal, frontal, trochlear, oculomotor (superior and inferior branches), nasocillary and abducens nerves. It also contains the superior ophthalmic vein. The inferior orbital fissure contains the inferior ophthalmic vein and infra-orbital artery and nerve.

Q15: B

The Association of Anaesthetist's of Great Britain and Ireland (AAGBI) have produced a document regarding the relative safety of neuraxial blockade with various anticoagulant and antiplatelet agents in pregnant and non-pregnant populations. With this platelet count they would state that the patient is at normal risk of a complication.

Q16: E

The King's College criteria for the assessment of liver failure due to paracetamol includes parameters A, B, C and D but not E.

Q17: B

The Brommage score assesses motor function in the lower limbs when the patient has received neuraxial blockade. Grade 1 is free movement of the legs and feet, grade 2 is the ability to just flex knees with free movement of the feet, grade 3 is unable to flex knees but the ability to move and grade 4 is an inability to move the legs or feet.

Q18: A

The Difficult Airway Society (DAS) has produced guidance on the assessment of and possible techniques for managing the extubation of the high risk airway. In this example the airway has been secured with an endotracheal tube but there are many features to suggest that the airway will be lost on extubation. Therefore, exchanging for a laryngeal mask is incorrect as there is no guarantee that you can ventilate. Neither would extubating the patient on remifentanil be a safe option, as their airway may not remain patent. The airway exchange catheter could be an option but there is no guarantee that if emergency intubation was required that the exchange catheter would be able to direct a new endotracheal tube. As the pathology is likely to rapidly improve and the airway is currently secure, tracheostomy seems too invasive and runs the risks associated with tracheostomy and spreading the infection into the mediastinum. Therefore, the best options is to post- pone extubation until the pus and oedema have cleared.

Q19: D

The Parkland formula is used to assess the maintenance fluid requirements for a burns patient in the first 24 hours. It is calculated as: 4 x percentage area burnt x mass. In this example, that would mean 4 x 20 x 50, which equals 4000ml in 24 hours. The question asks for a mls/hr rate, which would be 167ml/hr.

Q20: D
Cardiac output significantly increases in pregnancy and as a result increases renal blood flow and glomerular filtration rate. This leads to increased urine production and creatinine clearance. However, renal tubular reabsorption decreases.

Q21: C
The Association of Anaesthetist's of Great Britain and Ireland (AAGBI) have produced a document regarding the management of suspected malignant hyperthermia (MH) under anaesthesia. All the proposed treatments are correct, except the use of a depolarising neuromuscular agent as the only available drug of this class is suxamethonium, which causes MH in susceptible individuals.

Q22: A
This question asks about antiplatelet activity, not anticoagulant activity, therefore fondaparinux is wrong as this is a factor Xa inhibitor. Tirofiban is a glycoprotein IIa-IIIb inhibitor that is administered intravenously. Aspirin works by inhibiting thromboxane A2 synthesis. This leaves clopidogrel and ticagrelor which both work on the ADP receptor of platelets. Unlike ticagrelor, clopidogrel is a prodrug that requires once daily administration.

Q23: A
The superficial peroneal nerve supplies sensation to the dorsal aspect of the foot and is blocked by infiltrating local anaesthesia across the plantar junction. The deep peroneal nerve supplies sensation to the web space between the great toe and adjacent toe and is blocked by infiltrating local anaesthetic medial to the dorsalis pedis pulse. The saphenous nerve is blocked by infiltrating local anaesthetic over the medial malleolus and supplies the medial aspect of the ankle. The

sural nerve supplies the lateral aspect of the foot and is blocked by injecting local anaesthesia between the lateral malleolus and Achilles tendon. Finally, the tibial nerve is blocked by infiltrating behind the tibial artery at the level of the ankle and supplies sensation to the dorsum of the foot.

Q24: D

- Mapleson A circuits require (in theory) only the patient's actual minute volume to prevent rebreathing in a spontaneously breathing patient, but 2.5 time the minute volume when being positively pressure ventilated.
- Mapleson B circuits are not routinely used in clinical practice as they are cumbersome.
- Mapleson C circuits are used mainly in resuscitation and transfer settings as they are compact and portable, but they are not particularly efficient for spontaneously breathing or ventilated patients.
- Mapleson D circuits are less efficient for the spontaneously breathing patient than the ventilated patient as outlined in this case.
- Mapleson E circuits are referred to as an Ayre's T-piece and are useful for patients recovering from anaesthesia, as the tubing acts as a reservoir of oxygen for spontaneous respiration. The addition of a bag with a hole forms a Mapleson F circuit (Jackson Rees modification), which is used in paediatrics.

Q25: C

The additive effects of gasses to make a total pressure is described by Dalton's law on partial pressures. Boyle's law states that pressure is inversely proportional to volume. Charles' law relates volume and temperature in a directly proportional fashion. The Guy-Lussac law states that pressure and temperature are directly proportional. The universal gas constant is a number used in some equations denoted as R and is 8.314 J/K/mol.

Q26: C

Prilocaine is a useful local anaesthetic when performing a Bier's block. Unfortunately, it oxidises the haemoglobin molecule from the ferrous to ferric state which impairs oxygen transport on haemoglobin molecules. The treatment is methyl blue which reduces the haemoglobin back to the ferrous form. A Bier's block is not located near the anatomical location of the phrenic nerve. Histamine release would cause a red discolouration.

Q27: D

Actracurium, ketamine and bupivocaine exhibit stereoisomerism not tautomerism. Midazolam and sodium thiopental demonstrate tautomerism (i.e. their molecular structure alters depending on the pH of the solution), but midazolam changes from ionised to un-ionised with increasing pH whereas sodium thiopental is ionised in an alkaline environment and becomes unionised with reducing pH.

Q28: A

This question requires you to utilise the Hagan-Poiseulle equation. Doubling the radius will increase flow 16 fold, as flow is directly proportional to the radius to the power 4. Halving the radius will reduce the flow rate, as would doubling the length of the tubing. Doubling the pressure gradient or halving the viscosity will increase flow rate, but not as much as doubling the radius.

Q29: D

The European Porphyria Network has a list of drugs which are safe, probably safe and not safe in anaesthesia. In the above example all the drugs are considered safe, except sodium thiopental.

Q30: B

This patient is hypernatraemic, which means SIADH and cerebral salt wasting syndrome are incorrect as they cause hyponatraemia. There is nothing normal about the physiology and blood test results. Diabetes insipidus can occur in head injury, intracerebral bleed and pituitary surgery and classically presents as per the case in question. Excess salt intake would give either a euvolaemic or hypervolaemic state.

Printed in Great Britain
by Amazon